DON HARRIS

DEATH *by* LETHAL INGESTION

A Self-Imposed Sentence for Dietary Disobedience

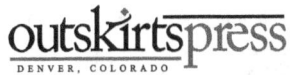

outskirtspress

DENVER, COLORADO

CONTENTS

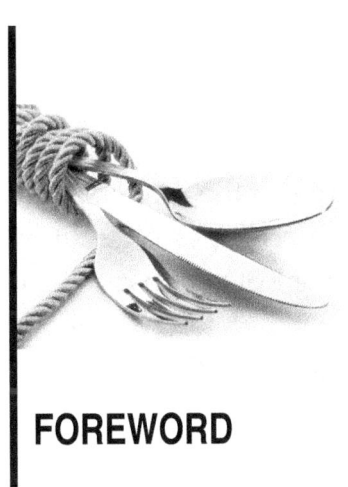

FOREWORD

Being fully aware of the standard protocol for the inclusion of a Foreword section in a published book, I have consciously decided not to follow that protocol for this work. There are two primary reasons for this decision. For this first and foundational project, which is based solely upon the Word of God, I felt strongly that any convincing of the readers' acceptance should be left to the Holy Spirit. The position I have taken is one of trying to avoid the standard 'marketing' practices used to authenticate and affirm an author's work. Such techniques certainly have their place and their value, so this is in no way an indictment of the millions of great published works that have been and will be produced using standard publishing protocol. In this instance, I regard myself as only a facilitator for the true author, the God of Abraham, Isaac, Jacob and the God of all of us who accept Him as Creator and Lord.

The reader will draw his/her own conclusions to that regard, particularly as it relates to my accuracy and thoroughness in the interpretation of the Word of God. The Bible has withstood many centuries of scrutiny and skepticism. As the fulfillment of prophesies, and time-tested principles within its pages have shown, there should be no question as to the truth of the Word itself.

The second reason for my break with standard protocol is in recognition of the fact this is a very controversial topic and I respect the potentially compromising position that anyone in the clergy or theological community may find themselves in if they choose to personally endorse this book. Of course, my hope for them or anyone else is that their commitment to obedience in whatever they accept as truth would cause them to act accordingly and responsibly, regardless of the consequences they might face.

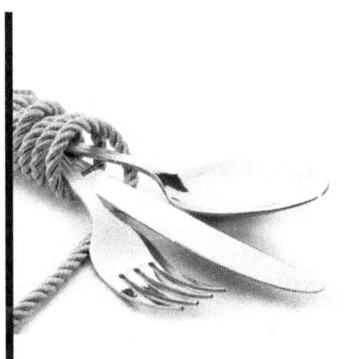

ACKNOWLEDGMENTS

The first recognition goes to the Holy Spirit, who inspired me to begin and has relentlessly prodded me to finish this book on this highly controversial topic. Thank you, Holy Spirit.

Secondly, I thank the various members of a small group ministry that has met in our home over the past several years. They shall remain nameless here because of my desire not to recognize some but overlook any one of them. That said, over the course of some of our group discussions, questions were raised about the Bible and what it has to say about foods that we should and should not eat, and related ordinances. The layout and content of this book is built around those questions.

I would also like to sincerely thank the many of my close friends and family and my Pastor, who have been so supportive and encouraging of my completing this project. You were instrumental in the motivation and accountability for me to keep going.

Many, many, thanks go to David & Cheryl Moore and Moore Xpressions Photography. You demonstrated the utmost in professionalism and excellence in producing my author photo. You have an undeniable gift from God that will undoubtedly come to be appreciated by many others in unimaginable ways!

Lastly, and most importantly, my deepest gratitude and appreciation goes to my beloved wife, Cynthia. Your support, encouragement and constructive criticism have been invaluable, not only to this project, but to me in all facets of our life together. You are truly a gift from God and an irreplaceable treasure!

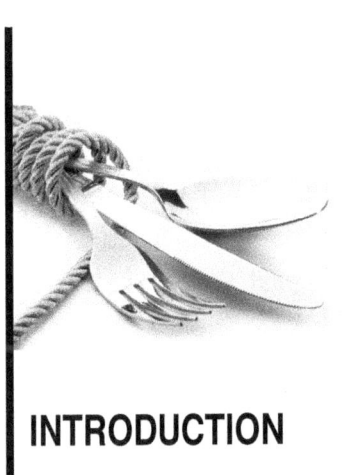

INTRODUCTION

Manufacturers of the finest automobiles in the world have strict standards for the care and feeding of the cars they produce. Many people spend thousands of dollars for rare breeds of animals for pets or for sport. They spend multiple thousands more to make sure that they are fed nothing but the best to make sure that "Fido" enjoys the best of health. Yet we neglect to do the same for, even abuse, our own bodies when it comes to what we eat – and we are supposed to be the most intelligent life on the planet!?!? Those expensive automobiles that are maintained so meticulously (some are even given names) come with Owner's Manuals that provide detailed information on how to maximize their useful life. Our "manufacturer", Almighty God, has provided us humans with a manual as well. It's called the Bible.

In the course of my life, there have been many tasks set before me that have been challenging, daunting, even intimidating. None have ever been more so than this one. After MUCH prayer and meditation, I have finally decided after several years of running away from the task, to move beyond the fear of public opinion and ridicule, in hopes that my obedience will positively affect someone else's life (perhaps even the lives of many) both physically and spiritually. I have spent many, many hours over the course of several years studying passages of scripture that are relevant to food. Much of it contradicts societal and cultural norms with regard to dietary choices. However, I am compelled to share what I have found.

I am reminded of something that I have said to my son and daughter several times over the years as they grew up. "I will gladly ruin your day if it means I will be saving your life." That is somewhat my sentiment here. I in no way want to offend with the material presented in this book, particularly since it is rooted in God's word. But, if it will save your life...

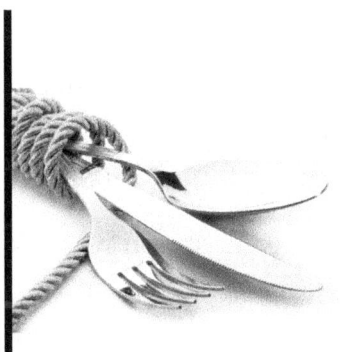

THE ALARM, THE INVITATION

Let me start out by being completely transparent. Having grown up in the south, I spent the first half of my life, thus far, deeply entrenched in its dietary traditions, sometimes even to the point of gluttony. In fact, I vividly recall a time as a young boy of about 14 years old attending a summer 4-H camp. At dinner, which was a barbecue, I devoured 3 half chickens, 9 hot dogs, a couple of burgers with beans, coleslaw and beverages all in one sitting! Overeating had sort of become my badge of honor and I was making my family proud!

I came from, what I learned later in life to be, a poor family. You sure couldn't tell that considering how we ate, though! I was particularly encouraged to over-eat by my immediate family through their praise and amazement at just how much I could eat. You would think that I would have been grossly obese with that kind of appetite, but the fact is, I went off to college at 6′4″ and 175 pounds. That stretched to a whopping 6′7″ and 203 pounds by the time I graduated college.

I should note that, much like most southerners, my family ate pork in some form or another at least once daily, but as many as three times on most days. It was common to have fatback for breakfast, pigs' feet or chitterlings (pig intestines) and rice for dinner. On other days, there was no shortage of other types of protein, like rabbit, raccoon, catfish, turtle and a host of others that I choose not to knowingly eat today. Little did I know, our menu content was in large part due to the fact that it was all my single-parent mother could afford. As the years went by, my bad dietary habits began to bear out their consequences in added pounds and rising blood pressure.

I have suffered a good deal of grief and sadness as I've seen close family members dying of cancer, heart attacks and complications of strokes and diabetes. More of the same continued to show itself in extended family, friends, co-workers and fellow church members. When the signs in my own body reached the point where I would literally get dizzy after a large meal, I knew that something had to change or I would be facing the same fate. Fortunately, this came at a time when I was seeking truth about some other issues in the Bible. As a result, I committed to study and sought to understand the heart of God on this matter of food choices. Cynthia and I walked through that process together and made some dramatic changes in our diet, and it has brought about some very positive changes in our health. We are on no prescription medications and have no lingering health problems. Thank you again, Lord! That process began some twenty-five years ago at the time of this writing. Sadly, the loss of health and life of those around me continues. I have since lost a brother to cancer and all three of my sisters suffer with high blood pressure. Two of them are obese and have diabetes as well.

We, particularly in America, are guilty of having traded the truth of God's Word for the lies of the enemy on so many fronts. This book deals specifically with the matter of our food choices. Those decisions, just as all choices we make, have consequences. In many cases, those consequences rob us of the very life of health and physical well-being that we would all hope for. Many of us knowingly reject or unwittingly overlook God's will for us to *"prosper and be in good health"* (3 John 1:2), and that He will *"heal all your diseases"* (Psalms 103:3). We fail to accept any personal responsibility for the bad decisions we make. Then, when the consequences of those decisions show up as cancer, diabetes, heart disease, high blood pressure or the like, we often simply pass it off as the inevitable "realities" of growing older. Nothing could be further from the truth! If we would only blow away that faulty thinking, originating from the father of lies, and replace it with standing on God's promises and the truth of His Word, we would be so much better off! This is something I believe down to the very core of my being. It has grown from what was my revelation to a personal experience and knowledge, from a desire to a passion for sharing this knowledge. In fact, it has come almost to the point of an obsession that consumes my thoughts and sometimes keeps me awake at night. Beginning several years ago, I found myself burdened with the call to sound the alarm: *We have violated the dietary laws of God, and imposed our own sentence by digging our graves with a knife and a fork!*

Now that I've got your attention, let me say that, other than the fact that I firmly believe God has called me to this task, my own grief and despair over count-less friends, church family, immediate and extended family members, either dead or dying of sickness and disease has compelled me to obey the mandate that I have been given. That is, to deliver the truth of God's word on this subject in a balanced and thorough, but uncompromised way so that anyone who reads and digests it (pun intended) will be able to make an in-formed decision about their own food choices for the rest of their lives on this planet. To that end, in an ef-fort to minimize questions of authenticity or opinion, no reference other than scripture is used to support the positions presented in this book. After all (assuming that you accept the Bible as the infallible truths from God), if God does not change (Malachi 3:6) and we are expected to accept His laws in totality (Matthew 5:18), the real task before all of us is to understand fully what He has tried to communicate to us through His word and to act according to our own personal convictions.

I would also challenge you to resist the temptation to put this book down and dismiss the content if it does not agree with your current beliefs about this topic of food. Digesting this information won't harm you at all. Instead, it just might make your life more abundant. After all, that is one of Jesus' personally expressed purposes in coming to us, that we might have life more abundantly. I think you would agree that a life with better health and fewer trips to the doctor, fewer medical bills and hospital stays leaves more room for greater enjoyment of the very precious life we have been given. We would be able to do more, experience more and give more. *He didn't come so we could have more "stuff", but more life!*

A fair question that you or any other person may have at this point is, **"Why should anyone care about what we eat or drink anyway? – What difference does it make?"** Unfortunately, that is a very common attitude, even amongst believers. To help you identify and overcome this thought process, consider this illustration:

I'm sure that you can think of at least one home or building other than your own that you are very familiar with. You love that place. It's beautiful! You really enjoy being there. You have attached very positive feelings to that place. You know the inside of it almost as well as the back of your hand – except for that one door, one room that you just never ventured to explore. You have every reason to believe that whatever is behind that door is every bit as pleasing as the rest of the building based on everything else you have seen there. Nevertheless, you've never made the effort to KNOW what lies behind that door. Maybe you have even taken a glimpse in passing, but quickly decided, 'ah, it's OK, but not as nice as the rest of the house' and you never went back.

The building I just described is symbolic of some parts of the Word of God, the Bible. Its words - *all of them* - are life to those who seek God and His truth. The 'room' I referred to is this largely overlooked, even avoided subject of dietary choices. For the most part, it is a door in the building that never gets opened in Christianity. On rare occasions, it is perused in passing, perhaps during a 'read through the Bible' campaign, but no real time or depth of study is spent there. Does that in any way diminish its value in God's overall plan? Absolutely not! As the Word says, ***all scripture is inspired by God and fit for our instruction.*** This particular subject is so often avoided and even rejected because it is in direct opposition to our own personally held beliefs and cultural norms.

My wife, Cynthia, and I have led and hosted a small group ministry in our home for several years and broached this subject, with their approval, as part of our time together. In setting up for the study, I thought it wise to first find out from the members of the group what questions they felt would need to be answered in order to be able to arrive at some reasonable conclusions to this potentially confusing and somewhat controversial subject. This writing is largely organized around the questions that arose out of those discussions. My thanks go to all of them for their contributions. Above all, thanks to God for giving me the grace to still carry out this task, despite my years of procrastination and intimidation.

Finally, it is my hope, prayer, belief and firm expectation that many lives will be made more abundant as a result of their repentance and obedience to God's commands, not only as it relates to food, but to all other aspects of life.

I am fully convinced that the Bible is the infallible, inspired Word of God. As such, its commands, precepts and instructions for holy living should be sought, understood and followed. Obviously, then, it is a given that the reader of this material must share that fundamental belief to add any real value to the time spent reading it. Beyond that, the age old important question is, *how will you respond if you learn that what you have been doing for much of your life is not acceptable in the eyes of God and may be literally killing you?* Will you change, or will you dismiss what you have learned and rationalize that it's OK to continue in your old ways? Will you keep the attitude that since you've done it this long and you're still here, why change now? There are also far too many who have the mindset of, "we're all going to die from something. So, what's the point of worrying about it? I'll just eat whatever I want and enjoy every bit of it until my time is up."

The answer to these questions is more important than you might first think. After all, the very essence of what repentance is comes to the forefront when we give it just a little thought. **When we *learn* better, we are expected to change our ways and *do* better.**

Please, now approach this material with an open mind *and an open Bible*. Lay aside any preconceptions you may have about dietary laws and allow the Holy Spirit to reveal the truth to you. Then, exercise one of the greatest gifts the Father has given you – the freedom to choose how you will respond. Of course, the greatest of gifts we were given is that of God's only son, Jesus, who sacrificed himself for our sins. Yet, even with that, out of His great love for us, He allows us to choose whether to accept that very precious gift. I believe that God is much more pleased when we willingly choose to follow Jesus rather than being forced. In the same way, we earthly fathers rejoice when our children make right decisions because they choose to, not simply because they are being compelled by rules or by force. God, through His boundless grace, leaves us to choose the extent of our commitment and obedience to His dietary laws and, for that matter, any of His commandments. However, in exercising our (believers') freedom, we must be ever mindful that **there will always be consequences that follow our actions, whether those actions are right or wrong.**

Realizing the very serious consequences of false teaching and misleading God's people, I have made every effort to 'rightly divide the Word of Truth'. If you invest the time to read through to the end, the choice of how to respond is yours. Choose wisely and you will be blessed whether my position is right or wrong. If right, I am blessed as well. If wrong, I am accountable and at God's mercy. May the Holy Spirit be with you as you read and, hopefully, study this material. Finally, may this information be a blessing to you and your loved ones.

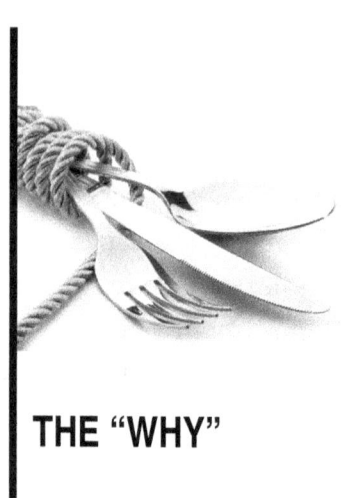

THE "WHY"

God created us as three dimensional beings – body, mind (soul) and spirit. As Christians, instructional emphasis is heavily skewed toward the spiritual aspect. I would even go so far as to say that many people believe that adherence to teaching about the final destination of the soul is the only thing that really matters from an eternal perspective. That is simply not the case. The reality is that it takes proper focus and attention to all three to assure the well-being of the whole person. The Word of God thoroughly addresses all of them. On the other hand, the church community seems, at the very least, to be out of balance in this regard. In setting forth the expectations for those who would be called the people of God, He commands us to be careful to follow all of His commandments, precepts and laws, as spelled out in the Books of the Law (the first five books of the Bible). The dietary laws are firmly embedded within those books and are as equally worth our attention and adherence as are the Ten Commandments, which are quite familiar to most of us. Many of us have memorized them since childhood.

The purpose of this writing is twofold. The first objective is to make an effort to direct some focus toward how we care for (feed, in particular) our physical bodies and how that relates to our overall spiritual health. Secondly, the hope is to break the continuing cycle of disease and premature deaths associated with dietary disobedience.

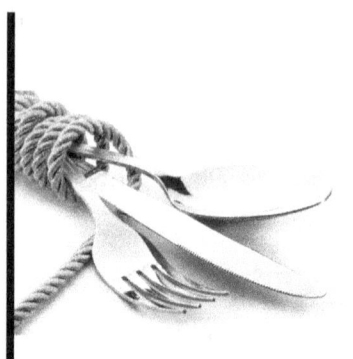

CLEAN VS. UNCLEAN

Of course, the basis for the pivotal questions about dietary considerations stems from two of the "*Books of Moses*", Leviticus 11 and its repetition in Deuteronomy 14. (The reference to Moses is deliberately highlighted here because that will be important to establish a key point later.) It is important to read and comprehend these passages in order to intelligently balance them against other Old Testament and later New Testament passages that must also be considered. The following is the account of scripture in its entirety as it is presented in the New International Version:

Leviticus 11

Clean and Unclean Food

> *1 The LORD said to Moses and Aaron, 2 "Say to the Israelites: 'Of all the animals that*

live on land, these are the ones you may eat: 3
You may eat any animal that has a split hoof
completely divided and that chews the cud.

4 " 'There are some that only chew the cud
or only have a split hoof, but you must not
eat them. The camel, though it chews the cud,
does not have a split hoof; it is ceremonial-
ly unclean for you. 5 The coney, [a] *though*
it chews the cud, does not have a split hoof;
it is unclean for you. 6 The rabbit, though it
chews the cud, does not have a split hoof; it is
unclean for you. 7 And the pig, though it has
a split hoof completely divided, does not chew
the cud; it is unclean for you. 8 You must not
eat their meat or touch their carcasses; they
are unclean for you.

Taking further insight into those land
animals that are identified as clean, they
have some key common characteristics.
They chew cud, which is regurgitated
food, to further break it down and remove toxins before passing it on to their
digestive system. There, nutrients are
extracted and the waste is then passed
along to the intestinal system. These animals also share in common that they do
not naturally feed on other animals as
prey or otherwise. Unclean animals, by

contrast, do not share those attributes. They are either predators, scavengers or whose bodies do not sufficiently remove toxins that render their flesh to be unfit for human consumption.

9 " 'Of all the creatures living in the water of the seas and the streams, you may eat any that have fins and scales. 10 But all creatures in the seas or streams that do not have fins and scales – whether among all the swarming things or among all the other living creatures in the water – you are to detest. 11 And since you are to detest them, you must not eat their meat and you must detest their carcasses. 12 Anything living in the water that does not have fins and scales is to be detestable to you.

As with the land animals, we find that the same commonalities exist among creatures living in the water as well as those in the following verses that are winged creatures. Those designated by God as clean are not predators or scavengers and the unclean are creatures of prey, scavengers or whose bodies do not expel, but are instead collectors of waste.

God's lists of those on land, in the waters or those that fly are not exhaustive, but are complete enough to provide us with clear guidelines to know what is or is not fit for our consumption. When you really think about it, this is just one more of the many ways that our heavenly Father demonstrates his love for us. He does this for our protection and promises that it will go well with us if we would only obey.

> 13 " 'These are the birds you are to detest and not eat because they are detestable: the eagle, the vulture, the black vulture, 14 the red kite, any kind of black kite, 15 any kind of raven, 16 the horned owl, the screech owl, the gull, any kind of hawk, 17 the little owl, the cormorant, the great owl, 18 the white owl, the desert owl, the osprey, 19 the stork, any kind of heron, the hoopoe and the bat. [b]

> 20 " 'All flying insects that walk on all fours are to be detestable to you. 21 There are, however, some winged creatures that walk on all fours that you may eat: those that have jointed legs for hopping on the ground. 22 Of these you may eat any kind of locust, katydid, cricket or grasshopper. 23 But all other winged creatures that have four legs you are to detest.

> 24 " 'You will make yourselves unclean by these; whoever touches their carcasses will be unclean till evening. 25 Whoever picks up one of their carcasses must wash his clothes, and he will be unclean till evening.

26 " 'Every animal that has a split hoof not completely divided or that does not chew the cud is unclean for you; whoever touches the carcass of any of them will be unclean. 27 Of all the animals that walk on all fours, those that walk on their paws are unclean for you; whoever touches their carcasses will be unclean till evening. 28 Anyone who picks up their carcasses must wash his clothes, and he will be unclean till evening. They are unclean for you.

29 " 'Of the animals that move about on the ground, these are unclean for you: the weasel, the rat, any kind of great lizard, 30 the gecko, the monitor lizard, the wall lizard, the skink and the chameleon. 31 Of all those that move along the ground, these are unclean for you. Whoever touches them when they are dead will be unclean till evening. 32 When one of them dies and falls on something, that article, whatever its use, will be unclean, whether it is made of wood, cloth, hide or sackcloth. Put it in water; it will be unclean till evening, and then it will be clean. 33 If one of them falls into a clay pot, everything in it will be unclean, and you must break the pot. 34 Any food that could be eaten but has water on it from such a pot is unclean, and any liquid that could be drunk from it is unclean. 35 Anything that one of their carcasses falls on becomes unclean; an oven or cooking pot must be broken up. They are unclean, and you are to regard them as unclean. 36 A spring, however, or a cistern for collecting water remains clean, but anyone who touches one of these carcasses is unclean. 37 If a carcass falls on any seeds that are to be planted, they remain clean. 38 But if water has been put on the seed and a carcass falls on it, it is unclean for you. 39 " 'If an animal that you are allowed to eat dies, anyone who touches the carcass will be unclean till evening. 40 Anyone who eats some of the carcass must wash his clothes, and he will be unclean till evening. Anyone who picks up the carcass must wash his clothes, and he will be unclean till evening.

41 " 'Every creature that moves about on the ground is detestable; it is not to be eaten. 42 You are not to eat any creature that moves about on the ground, whether it moves on its belly or walks on all fours or on many feet; it is detestable. 43 Do not defile yourselves by any of these creatures. Do not make yourselves unclean by means of them or be made unclean by them. 44 I am the LORD your

*God; consecrate yourselves and be holy, because I am holy. Do not make yourselves unclean by any creature that moves about on the ground. 45 I am the LORD who brought you up out of Egypt to be your God; therefore **be holy**, because I am holy.*

*46 " 'These are the regulations concerning animals, birds, every living thing that moves in the water and every creature that moves about on the ground. 47 **You must distinguish between the unclean and the clean**, between living creatures that may be eaten and those that may not be eaten.' "*

We find this set of dietary instructions repeated in Deuteronomy 14, which I will not repeat here, although it would certainly be beneficial for your learning and retention to read it directly from the Bible. The fact that God was so detailed and specific in giving these instructions to His people and the fact that He repeated it so explicitly, strongly suggests how important it was (and is) to Him. Obviously, many of us look at most of this as 'irrelevant' for us in our day and time. For example, most of us would never even consider taking 'road kill' (Deuteronomy 14:21) as food! This is where we need to apply the common sense realization that God was speaking to His people *at that time* in language that they well understood. Our task and challenge is to seek the wisdom to determine what, if any, of all of this is pertinent to us *today*. That will become clearer as we now address the questions (fair questions) that our small group raised. I anticipate that you, the reader, may have many of the same questions.

You will likely note that some of the scripture passages referenced are somewhat lengthy. This is by intent. As I perused just some of the myriad of materials, books and articles produced on this subject, I reached the conclusion that most, if not all, of the misinformation found is a result of what I would call the "microwave syndrome".

We have become so accustomed, in our age of convenience, to getting everything that we want instantaneously, that we are often guilty of that same mindset when it comes to seeking the Word of God for answers to life's questions. As such, we look for just the right *little* verse that will give us that "Ah hah!!!" moment. As a result, too many times, we don't read far enough beyond or ahead of that precious little morsel of wisdom to get the complete picture of what our loving heavenly Father wanted to convey. He admonishes us to read, study and *meditate* on the Word. The latter, meditate, allows the Holy Spirit to do as the Bible says – "teach us all things". When we are patient and allow time for information that we must make decisions about to "marinate" in our spirit, it is amazing how the Holy Spirit will quietly but clearly reveal the truth to us.

I must admit that there is another reason why I include the full context of the Bible references. It is also quite likely that some readers (certainly not you, though!) will not actually take the time to keep a Bible alongside while reading this and actually read the full passages, so I find it more convenient to include them here. Now, with all that said, let's proceed further into the subject at hand.

Prior to delving into the biblical challenges to the Old Testament dietary laws, it may be beneficial to establish some logic as to why some of "God's creatures" are regarded as 'unclean' anyway. For that we must go back to Genesis.

When God instructed Noah regarding who and what to take into the ark with him before the great flood, He told him to take seven pairs of every *'clean'* animal and two pairs of every *'unclean'* animal (Genesis 7:1-6). If they were unclean, why did God want them preserved anyhow? With some thought, the answer is relatively simple. God wanted to maintain the balance of nature that was very important to the preservation and maintenance of the planet. Whether in earth, sky or sea, **there must be an appropriate balance of clean creatures and scavengers. Yes, scavengers!** God created an environment that was originally intended to be self-maintaining. (Remember that before Adam and Eve ate of the forbidden fruit, it was God's plan that Adam was not going to have to work (toil), but to simply enjoy the fruit from the beautiful garden that God had created and for Adam and Eve to commune daily with Him.)

Of course, God and Noah knew that the flood would end and life would start all over again. If the beauty and health of the planet were to be restored and maintained, there would still need to be those creatures which, by nature, would clean up the waste left behind by all the others. That includes cleaning up after us humans. (Have you ever wondered how Noah and his family survived without sickness while stuck in the ark with all those animals for 40 days? Hmmm!!!)

Let me share a simple example: It is highly likely that you may have observed a lake or pond as something that was very pleasant to see as you passed by it. It may even have been a favored little fishing spot at one time. However, as the years passed, it became disgustingly algae infested and putrid! That is because there was a shortage of bottom feeders to keep the water filtered and suitable for any top feeders that might have been present. Unfortunately, catfish (bottom feeders) are a favored fresh water treat for many people and are joyfully hauled out, dressed, seasoned, battered, fried and savored to the very last morsel. The problem with this is, God says (with them not having both fins and scales) **they were never intended to be for food, despite the fact that they taste so good!** Multiply that by the nets full of crabs, lobsters, shrimp, mollusks and other bottom feeders hauled out of the earth's waters every day to meet the demands of seafood lovers who crave those delectable treats. Yes, I did call them delectable! Remember that I enjoyed the same for many years of my life and have no room to be judgmental of those who still do. Yet, I feel that I have learned better and am compelled to teach as many as will give ear to learn and do likewise, in keeping with **Philippians 3:16-19,** *"Only let us live up to what we have already attained. Join with others in following my example, brothers and take note of those who live according to the pattern we gave you. For, as I have often told you before and now say again even with tears, many live as enemies of the cross of Christ. Their destiny is destruction, <u>their god is their stomach,</u> and their glory is in their shame".*

The point is, just because something tastes so good, that is not reason enough to safely regard it as acceptable food – not any more than obvious acts of sin, like sex outside of marriage, substance abuse and the like (which may be quite pleasurable for the moment) are righteous in the sight of God. As we all know, they are not!

God clearly gave us instruction in righteous living and spelled out in great detail what is sin and He commands our obedience. At the same time, He knows that his people love to eat and offered this promise in

Isaiah 1:19, *"if you are willing and obedient, you will eat the best from the land".*

This brings us closer to the questions at hand: How does what we choose to eat fit into all of this and what else does God have to say about it beyond the old Mosaic laws?

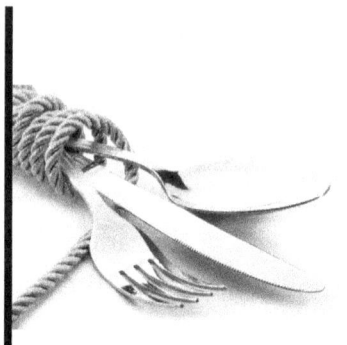

OLD TESTAMENT, NEW TESTAMENT

What about New Testament scriptures that *appear* to nullify the Old Testament teachings . . . e.g., only blood and food sacrificed to idols is forbidden and "eat anything sold in the meat market"?

OK, let's just admit it. Most of us Christians are more comfortable with the New Testament scriptures. We would just as soon dispense with all that Old Testament stuff anyway. After all, didn't Christ 'nail all that to the cross' when He became the supreme sacrifice for our sins? I'm hanging my eternal hat on a big NO! **What Jesus canceled was the *curse* of the law of sin and death (you sin, you die – the debt of death).** Through faith in Him, asking for forgiveness and (the part we don't like – changing our ways) repentance, we no longer have to be subject to the penalty for our sins, whatever they may be. The penalty for sin, which we all are subject to, is death. But praise God!!! Jesus paid the price for every one of us with one selfless act – dying on the cross. Throughout the Bible, the recurring theme is rebellion and redemption. The identification of rebellion is tied to the foundational laws that God set forth in the Old Testament and none of the laws or principles they represent have changed. Even the penalty remains the same as it always was. Eternal death still awaits those who reject the free gift of salvation that is available to all who willingly accept it. Only the remediation for violating them has changed.

Jesus, himself, said *"Do not think that I have come to abolish the Law or the Prophets. I have come not to abolish them but to fulfill them."* (Matt. 5:17)

Scripture teaches us that **Jesus was in every way a Jew and lived according to the Way God outlined for His people. We would have to then assume that Jesus' dietary practices followed God's laws regarding the same.** In fact, that is somewhat confirmed in the account of Peter's vision in Acts 10:9-16. Peter's response to being told to eat all sorts of what was regarded as forbidden foods was *"Surely not, Lord! I have never eaten anything impure or unclean!"* That emphatic statement by Peter strongly suggests that this was a total taboo, not only to Peter, but to Jesus as well.

A voice from heaven replied to Peter (verse 15), *"Do not call anything impure that God has made clean."* This is one of those proverbial "Ah Ha!!!" verses referenced as proof that anything goes as acceptable food. After all, God, Himself, pronounced them as clean in that verse – or did he? To find the answer, we must do as I suggested earlier. We need to read before and after verses 9-16 to see the full picture of what was really happening here. At the beginning of the chapter, in verses 1-8, we see that at the very same time that God was speaking to Peter through a vision, He was also working on Cornelius, an Italian centurion – a non-Jew – also in a vision, through the voice of an angel. The passage reads:

> *[1]At Caesarea there was a man named Cornelius, a centurion in what was known as the Italian Regiment. [2]He and all his family were devout and God-fearing; he gave generously to those in need and prayed to God regularly. [3]One day at about three in the afternoon he had a vision. He distinctly saw an angel of God, who came to him and said, "Cornelius!" [4]Cornelius stared at him in fear. "What is it, Lord?" he asked. The angel answered, "Your prayers and gifts to the poor have come up as a memorial offering before God. [5]Now send men to Joppa to bring back a man named Simon who is called Peter. [6]He is*

staying with Simon the tanner, whose house is by the sea." ⁷When the angel who spoke to him had gone, Cornelius called two of his servants and a devout soldier who was one of his attendants. ⁸He told them everything that had happened and sent them to Joppa.

Now, let's take a look at what comes after verse 16 of the same chapter (Acts 10).

¹⁷While Peter was wondering about the meaning of the vision, the men sent by Cornelius found out where Simon's house was and stopped at the gate. ¹⁸They called out, asking if Simon who was known as Peter was staying there. ¹⁹While Peter was still thinking about the vision, the Spirit said to him, "Simon, three[a] men are looking for you. ²⁰So get up and go downstairs. Do not hesitate to go with them, for I have sent them." ²¹Peter went down and said to the men, "I'm the one you're looking for. Why have you come?" ²²The men replied, "We have come from Cornelius the centurion. He is a righteous and God-fearing man, who is respected by all the Jewish people. A holy angel told him to have you come to his house so that he could hear what you have to say." ²³Then Peter invited the men into the house to be his guests....

How mysteriously God works! The link is completed. God sent an angel to speak to a non-Jewish, devout, God-fearing man (Cornelius) to seek out Peter, a Jewish Christian, to begin the spread of the gospel to the Gentiles. Prior to this, a Jew would not want to be caught dead in the home of a Gentile! So you see, it becomes *apparent* that Peter's vision was not really about a sudden cleansing of food that was formerly declared unclean, even detestable, but God's way of using a set of laws profoundly entrenched in the fabric of the lives of His people to tear down the walls that would begin the process of opening the doors for you and me to be able to hear the same gospel some 2,000 years later. But, wait. I must be fair. That is mere supposition at this point. We must be ever so careful not to add (or take away from) scripture to support any position we want to promote. We need something more conclusive. For that, we must read further:

> "....*The next day Peter started out with them, and some of the brothers from Joppa went along.* [24]*The following day he arrived in Caesarea. Cornelius was expecting them and had called together his relatives and close friends.* [25]*As Peter entered the house, Cornelius met him and fell at his feet in reverence.* [26]*But Peter made him get up. "Stand up," he said, "I am only a man myself."* [27]*Talking with him, Peter went inside and*

found a large gathering of people. ²⁸*He said to them: "You are well aware that it is against our law for a Jew to associate with a Gentile or visit him. But God has shown me that I should not call any* <u>man</u> *impure or unclean.* ²⁹*So when I was sent for, I came without raising any objection. May I ask why you sent for me?"* ³⁰*Cornelius answered: "Four days ago I was in my house praying at this hour, at three in the afternoon. Suddenly a man in shining clothes stood before me* ³¹*and said, 'Cornelius, God has heard your prayer and remembered your gifts to the poor.* ³²*Send to Joppa for Simon, who is called Peter. He is a guest in the home of Simon the tanner, who lives by the sea.'* ³³*So I sent for you immediately, and it was good of you to come. Now we are all here in the presence of God to listen to everything the Lord has commanded you to tell us."*

³⁴*Then Peter began to speak: "I now realize how true it is that God does not show favoritism* ³⁵*but accepts* <u>men</u> *from every nation who fear him and do what is right.* ³⁶*You know the message God sent to the people of Israel, telling the good news of peace through Jesus Christ, who is Lord of all.* ³⁷*You know what has happened throughout Judea, beginning in*

Galilee after the baptism that John preached – [38]how God anointed Jesus of Nazareth with the Holy Spirit and power, and how he went around doing good and healing all who were under the power of the devil, because God was with him. [39]"We are witnesses of everything he did in the country of the Jews and in Jerusalem. They killed him by hanging him on a tree, [40]but God raised him from the dead on the third day and caused him to be seen. [41]He was not seen by all the people, but by witnesses whom God had already chosen – by us who ate and drank with him after he rose from the dead. [42]He commanded us to preach to the people and to testify that he is the one whom God appointed as judge of the living and the dead. [43]All the prophets testify about him that everyone who believes in him receives forgiveness of sins through his name."

[44]While Peter was still speaking these words, the Holy Spirit came on all who heard the message. [45]The circumcised believers who had come with Peter were astonished that the gift of the Holy Spirit had been poured out even on the Gentiles. [46]For they heard them speaking in tongues[b] and praising God. Then Peter said, [47]"Can anyone keep these people from being baptized with water? They have received the Holy Spirit just as we have."

⁴⁸So he ordered that they be baptized in the name of Jesus Christ. Then they asked Peter to stay with them for a few days.

So, we see more clearly that Peter's vision was not literally about food at all, but was used to open the door for the spreading of the gospel. But, to solidify the point further, **the evidence becomes even more conclusive when Peter has to explain the visit to Cornelius' home to his inner circle and other believers.** Let's continue:

Acts 11

Peter Explains His Actions

¹The apostles and the brothers throughout Judea heard that the Gentiles also had received the word of God. ²So when Peter went up to Jerusalem, the circumcised believers criticized him ³and said, "You went into the house of uncircumcised men and ate with them." ⁴Peter began and explained everything to them precisely as it had happened: ⁵"I was in the city of Joppa praying, and in a trance I saw a vision. I saw something like a large sheet being let down from heaven by its four corners, and it came down to where I was. ⁶I looked into it and saw four-footed animals of the earth, wild beasts, reptiles, and birds of the air. ⁷Then I heard a voice telling me, 'Get up, Peter. Kill and eat.' ⁸"I replied, 'Surely not, Lord! Nothing impure or unclean has ever entered my mouth.' ⁹"The voice spoke from heaven a second time, 'Do not call anything impure that God has made clean.' ¹⁰This happened three times, and then it was all pulled up to heaven again. ¹¹"Right then three men who had been sent to me from Caesarea stopped at the house where I was staying. ¹²The Spirit told me to have no hesitation about going with them. These six brothers also went with me, and we entered the man's house. ¹³He told us how he had seen an angel appear in his house and say, 'Send to Joppa for Simon who is called Peter. ¹⁴He will bring you a message through which you and all your household will be saved.' ¹⁵"As I began to speak, the Holy Spirit came on them as he had come on us at the beginning. ¹⁶Then I remembered what the Lord had said: 'John baptized with[a]water, but you will be baptized with the Holy Spirit.' ¹⁷**So if God gave them the same gift as he gave us, who believed in the Lord Jesus Christ, who was I to think that I could oppose God?"** ¹⁸When they heard this, they had no further objections and praised God, saying,

"So then, God has granted even the Gentiles repentance unto life."

Given this final account of his vision and subsequent actions, there should remain no question about the meaning and intent God had in mind. **Many, in their attempt to justify what they have been doing and continue to do with regard to violation of God's dietary laws, have referred to Acts 10: 15 as conclusive proof. However, when presented in its full context, that becomes quite a difficult position to defend.**

With that verse eliminated as a 'license to eat the pig', let's move to another that seems to support the notion of 'eat whatever you want and it's OK'. That would be Romans 14:14 where Paul says,

"14As one who is in the Lord Jesus, I am fully convinced that no food[b] is unclean in itself."

My first response to this is to remind you that God, at this point, had long since established, and it was well-entrenched into the culture of His people, just what was considered *'food'* and what was not. There is no need to repeat that here. Secondly, when we again 'zoom out' and take in the entire 14th chapter, we see that this discourse is not about what is to be considered as food as much as it addresses the centuries-old argument about eating meat versus eating only vegetables. Those from the vegan camp will often refer back to Genesis 1:29 to support their argument that vegetarianism was God's original intent for humanity. Therefore, it must be the best and preferred choice.

(*Then God said, "I give you every* **seed-bearing** *plant on the face of the whole earth and every tree that has fruit with seed in it. They will be yours for food."*).

Additional biblical evidence suggests otherwise, as you will see from further reading. Let's now take a look at the whole chapter of Romans 14.

The Weak and the Strong

> [1]*Accept him whose faith is weak, without passing judgment on disputable matters.* [2]*One <u>man's faith allows him to eat every-thing, but another man, whose faith is weak, eats only vegetables.</u>* We will see as we read on that 'everything' really means 'meat as well as vegetables. [3]*The man who eats everything must not look down on him who does not, and the man who does not eat everything must not condemn the man who does, for God has accepted him.* [4]*Who are you to judge someone else's servant? To his own master he stands or falls. And he will stand, for the Lord is able to make him stand.* [5]*One man considers one day more sacred than another; another man considers every day alike. Each one should be fully convinced in his*

own mind. [6]He who regards one day as special, does so to the Lord. **He who eats meat, eats to the Lord, for he gives thanks to God; and he who abstains, does so to the Lord and gives thanks to God.** *[7]For none of us lives to himself alone and none of us dies to himself alone. [8]If we live, we live to the Lord; and if we die, we die to the Lord. So, whether we live or die, we belong to the Lord. [9]For this very reason, Christ died and returned to life so that he might be the Lord of both the dead and the living. [10]You, then, why do you judge your brother? Or why do you look down on your brother? For we will all stand before God's judgment seat. [11]It is written: " 'As surely as I live,' says the Lord, 'every knee will bow before me; every tongue will confess to God.' "[a] [12]So then, each of us will give an account of himself to God. [13]Therefore let us stop passing judgment on one another. Instead, make up your mind not to put any stumbling block or obstacle in your brother's way. [14]As one who is in the Lord Jesus, I am fully convinced that no food[b] is unclean in itself. But if anyone regards something as unclean, then for him it is unclean. [15]If your brother is distressed because of what you eat, you are no longer acting in love. Do not by your eating destroy your brother for* *whom Christ died. *[16]*Do not allow what you consider good to be spoken of as evil. *[17]*For the kingdom of God is not a matter of eating and drinking, but of righteousness, peace and joy in the Holy Spirit, *[18]*because anyone who serves Christ in this way is pleasing to God and approved by men. *[19]*Let us therefore make every effort to do what leads to peace and to mutual edification. *[20]***Do not destroy the work of God for the sake of food. All food is clean, but it is wrong for a man to eat anything that causes someone else to stumble. **[21]***It is better not to eat meat or drink wine or to do anything else that will cause your brother to fall. **[22]***So whatever you believe about these things keep between yourself and God.** *Blessed is the man who does not condemn himself by what he approves. *[23]*But the man who has doubts is condemned if he eats, because his eating is not from faith; and everything that does not come from faith is sin.*

We see clearly in verse 21 that Paul was referring to meat and wine, both of which were very much accepted amongst God's people of the day, yet there was obviously a strong contingent of immature Christians who believed that they should adhere to what they believed was God's original intent going back to the

Garden of Eden – a complete and totally vegetarian diet. In fact, **there are still many today who insist that the key to healthy living is to return to the so called Eden diet. Let's dispense with that very quickly.**

Immediately following the account of the Garden of Eden and Adam and Eve's eviction, comes the account of Cain and Abel that we are all so familiar with (Genesis 4:1-5). Even that early in human history, God unquestionably establishes the acceptability of meat from Abel's flocks as food.

Incidentally, I'm going to take this opportunity to digress just a little. There has been much speculation as to why God accepted Abel's offering and rejected Cain's. I will weigh in and render my own position. I think we too often look so deeply for some spiritual insight that we overlook the obvious. It's right in the scripture! In verse 3, we read that Cain brought *an* offering. In verse 4, we see that Abel brought forth out of the *firstfruits* of his flocks as an offering to God. God was establishing the principle of tithing at the very beginning of human history. He wants the *first* of our increase, not just *some* of what we have left over after taking what we want! Ahhhh!!! It felt good getting that off my chest, now back to the subject . . .

The next New Testament verse that we will examine is found in 1 Corinthians 10:25, where it says, *"Eat anything sold in the meat market without raising questions of conscience."* Many believers have said something to the effect of "There it is! That's the ticket! After all, right there in the Bible – it did say **anything**, didn't it!!! Not so fast, hold the fork! I have two points to make. At the risk of being repetitive, we must look at the verse in light of its full scriptural context. When we do so, we find that this was a statement made in the midst of a teaching about partaking of food sacrificed to idols, which is a part of pagan worship. Paul teaches that although we have certain freedoms as believers, it is not always prudent to exercise that freedom. We must not only think of ourselves, but also about non-believers who might eventually become saved. We must also be considerate of less mature Christians who may not yet fully understand enough about the "Way" to discern freedom of choice from overt sin or disobedience.

The second point I would make requires some common sense logic and application of what we have already learned. We must consider the Lord's detailed regulations, laws and commands about clean and unclean foods, and the fact that this was coming from a Jewish believer (Paul), spoken to other Jewish believers. We should also understand and assume that *"anything sold in the meat market"* would not include ham, pork chops, bacon, shrimp, lobsters or oysters on the half-shell.

While we're in the passage (see below), let's take a look at yet another verse that is referenced as an

open license to partake of whatever our hearts desire,
Verse 27. *". . . eat whatever is put before you without raising questions of conscience"*. Note that the first part of
the same verse says, "If an **unbeliever** invites you to
a meal ..." This, again, is not an open license to disregard God's established dietary laws. **He extends His
grace for those exceptional occasions when our wit-
ness is more important than our religion.** He would
not want our strict adherence to His laws to be offen-
sive to someone who is simply extending hospitality
to a fellow human being and who doesn't have a clue
about God's Ways regarding food choices, in particular. To the contrary, the door should be left open to
share the gospel of Christ as Lord and savior rather
than slammed shut because of our spiritual arrogance
and insensitivity. However, we must be mindful that
this extension of grace is meant to be the exception and
not the rule. It should almost go without saying, but
we should also not assume that verse 27 grants license
for *believers* to willingly and frequently gather together
at a feast that includes unclean meat. The expectation
from God is quite to the contrary. We are (or are supposed to be) students of His Word and should know
better. The real problem that we have, though, is not
one of being unaware of what the Bible says. **We more
often want to alter the interpretation of what we read
to validate what we do rather than conform our ways
to His ways!** This fact is by no means limited to dietary
choices. We are all likely guilty of taking a tidbit of

scripture (often out of context) and twisting its meaning to legitimize our wrongful actions. However, we should be ever mindful that no matter how successful we are at fooling others and maybe even ourselves, *"Be not deceived.*

God is not mocked." The latter part of John 10:35 serves as a reminder to us that the Word of God cannot be broken, but will stand on its own. Instead, we more likely break ourselves over it. A line from an old secular hit song comes to mind and perfectly expresses this truth when I think about it: **"I fought the law and the law won."**

The Believer's Freedom

> [23]*"Everything is permissible" – but not everything is beneficial. "Everything is permissible" – but not everything is constructive.* [24]*Nobody should seek his own good, but the good of others.* [25]*Eat anything sold in the meat market without raising questions of conscience,* [26]*for, "The earth is the Lord's, and everything in it."*[c] [27]*If some unbeliever invites you to a meal and you want to go, eat whatever is put before you without raising questions of conscience.* [28]*But if anyone says to you,*

"This has been offered in sacrifice," then do not eat it, both for the sake of the man who told you and for conscience' sake[d] — 29the other man's conscience, I mean, not yours. For why should my freedom be judged by another's conscience? 30If I take part in the meal with thankfulness, why am I denounced because of something I thank God for? 31So whether you eat or drink or whatever you do, do it all for the glory of God. 32Do not cause anyone to stumble, whether Jews, Greeks or the church of God — 33even as I try to please everybody in every way. For I am not seeking my own good but the good of many, so that they may be saved.

Perhaps one of the most challenging passages to this idea that God's dietary laws from the Old Testament still stand as relevant today is found in Acts 15: 28-29, which reads, *"28It seemed good to the Holy Spirit and to us not to burden you with anything beyond the following requirements: 29You are to abstain from food sacrificed to idols, from blood, from the meat of strangled animals and from sexual immorality."*

This doesn't by any stretch of the imagination mean that it's open season on the baby back ribs any more than it means that murder, lying and stealing are OK as long as you are a Gentile Christian and not a Jew! At the risk of bordering on being absolutely absurd, I offer the following analogy: Picture in your mind a 45 year old man (who is not mentally challenged) dressed in a too little t-shirt and training pants, scrunched onto a tricycle, happily pedaling up and down his driveway. You ask him why he's doing that and he replies in a manner typical of a 3 year-old, "Daddy said if I don't wet my pants, learn how to talk good and ride my tricycle by myself, he would be happy." Of course, it is ludicrous to even think that a parent would literally mean that they would accept that their child's development would stop there! Those developmental milestones, successfully achieved, would be good indicators that the child had the foundational skills to go on and grow into a healthy, normal functioning adult. He would be well-prepared to go to school with other children and learn and develop as God has uniquely designed.

I sincerely hope that this 'nutty' example effectively helps to illustrate my point. Meeting the few requirements Paul laid out for early Gentile converts was just the beginning, laying a foundation that would be built upon later.

To fully understand this much *mis*understood passage, we need to back up a few verses to 19-21:

> [19]*"It is my judgment, therefore, that we should not make it difficult for the Gentiles who are **turning** to God.* [20]*Instead we should write to them, telling them to abstain from food polluted by idols, from sexual immorality, from*

the meat of strangled animals and from blood.
²¹For Moses has been preached in every city
from the earliest times and is read in the syn-
agogues on every Sabbath."

Notice the operative word "turn**ing**" in verse 19. The real message here is that Paul and Barnabus understood the fact that the entirety of God's prescribed plan for holy living was too much and too difficult for new converts to take in all at once, and further, that conversion is a process, not an event. The 'macro' issues of blood (because of potential blood-borne diseases), the meat of strangled animals (the flesh of the animals would be contaminated with the blood not having been allowed to be drained as God prescribed) and sexual immorality were merely *a good start* in the new walk of Gentile converts. The idea was that these new believers would eventually get the rest of what they needed to know about holy living as God's people because, as was stated in verse 21, *"Moses has been preached in every city from the earliest times and **is read in the synagogues on every Sabbath.**"* The commandments, dietary laws and laws regarding cleanliness, infectious diseases and the like were cloaked in the Mosaic scriptures. It was assumed and expected that these Gentile converts, including us, who earnestly seek God and study His word, as we attend regular church services, would eventually learn all that He has so intently preserved for our good. The collection of writings that we know of as the Bible has survived intact for thousands of years because that was and is God's plan. None of it is to be overlooked or disregarded and nothing is to be added to it. That includes His dietary instructions. It is not there simply for our reading pleasure or just to fill up the pages! It is for our growth and edification.

Sadly, too many churches have evolved to the point where the music and the message are a meticulously coordinated program designed to evoke an emotional response from the congregation that keeps them coming back and paying the bills to keep things running. These are both valuable and necessary, but are severely lacking if they are not supported by solid, fundamental Bible reading and instruction. The sad truth is, most regular churchgoers don't bring a Bible (in paper or electronic form) to church and read very little, if at all, at home. It is highly unlikely that a few songs, five points and a poem are enough to get and keep anyone firmly grounded in the ways of God.

Now, to continue with the scripture reference, having reached a consensus amongst the brothers in the faith, it was decided to communicate the following message to the Gentile believers:

The Council's Letter to Gentile Believers

The apostles and elders, your brothers, To the Gentile believers in Antioch, Syria and

Cilicia: Greetings. ²⁴We have heard that some went out from us without our authorization and disturbed you, troubling your minds by what they said. ²⁵So we all agreed to choose some men and send them to you with our dear friends Barnabas and Paul – ²⁶men who have risked their lives for the name of our Lord Jesus Christ. ²⁷Therefore we are sending Judas and Silas to confirm by word of mouth what we are writing. ²⁸It seemed good to the Holy Spirit and to us not to burden you with anything beyond the following requirements: ²⁹You are to abstain from food sacrificed to idols, from blood, from the meat of strangled animals and from sexual immorality. You will do well to avoid these things.

It is certainly easy to see how such a letter can be regarded as cancellation of the Mosaic dietary laws for Gentile Christians, but I believe the greater body of evidence supports otherwise.

1 Timothy 4

Instructions to Timothy

> *¹The Spirit clearly says that in later times some will abandon the faith and follow deceiving spirits and things taught by demons.*

> [2]*Such teachings come through hypocritical liars, whose consciences have been seared as with a hot iron.* [3]*They forbid people to marry and order them to* <u>abstain from certain foods</u>*, which God created to be received with thanksgiving by those who believe and who know the truth.* [4]*For everything God created is good, and nothing is to be rejected if it is received with thanksgiving,* [5]*because it is consecrated by the word of God and prayer.*

The above passage is obviously another that has been and will likely continue to be used to justify an 'anything goes' mentality toward what we eat. I, however, strongly believe that the scriptural evidence already presented supports otherwise. I, again, don't want to risk being guilty of adding to the Word, but previously addressed New Testament scriptures, when viewed in full context, specifically identified the argument about foods that should be abstained from as being about whether or not to include meat in the diet. Regarding the latter part of verse 3, "certain foods which God created to be received with thanksgiving . . .' note again the operative word, *foods*. That was not meant to be all inclusive, anything we want to stick in our mouth, but within the guidelines of what God had already defined and identified as *food*.

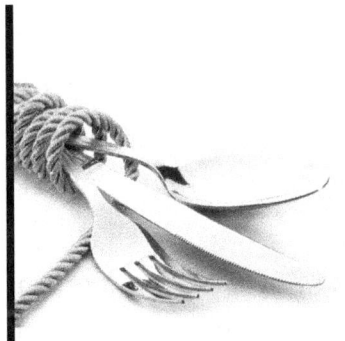

FOR JEWS ONLY OR ALL CHRISTIANS?

Isn't this stuff only for the Old Testament Jews and not necessarily for us today?

To answer this, let's start in the Old Testament, where God addresses the dietary and other regulations, but first, let me interject a statement for you to ponder as we go forward. There are numerous references in the Old Testament books of Deuteronomy, Joshua, I Samuel, I & II Kings that admonish the people of God to "walk in His ways" as described in the books of Moses. These included God's laws, commandments, decrees and precepts - rules for daily living. Why, then, would He take lightly or reverse positions on His own instructions as to how we are to take care of the Temple of the Holy Spirit - our bodies? **Why would God give such detailed instructions multiple times,** only to later decide, 'never mind, you don't really have to pay any attention to what I said before? It doesn't matter now!'

Going back to Deuteronomy 14:21, which we touched on earlier, it is fair and important to note that the remaining portion of the same verse presents an interesting thought. After admonishing His people not to eat anything found already dead, God instructed,

> *"You may give it to the foreigner residing in any of your towns, and they may eat it, or you may sell it to any other foreigner. But you are a people holy to the LORD YOUR GOD."*[(B)]

At this point, you are probably thinking something like, "Why would God say that? Isn't that cruel, maybe even hypocritical? Those are fair questions to ask for sure. But, I would pose another question to you in light of the latter part of that same verse. Why wouldn't we want to be regarded as among His "holy people" set apart as His special possession? Instead, we should recognize that this was one of many instances where God makes it clear that He only wants the best for His people.

When talking about the matter of eating fat and rare meat (meat with the blood still in it) God instructed Moses to tell the people, "Any Israelite *or any alien living among you* who eats any blood – I will set my face against that person …. and will cut him off from his people." (Lev. 17:10) Verse 12 of the same chapter continues: "Therefore I say to the Israelite, None of you may eat blood, nor may an alien living among you eat blood."

God addresses the same subject earlier in Leviticus, sending the message to his people, *"All the fat is the Lord's. This is a lasting ordinance for the generations to come, wherever you live: you must not eat fat or any blood."* (Lev. 3:16b-17)

These passages transcend both time and cultural norms. When God said *"wherever you live"* He took away the rationalization of "When in Rome, do as the Romans do." The Lord also included Gentiles when He said, *"any alien living among you"* (Lev. 17:12)

Let's also take a look at the 'fat' issue, briefly. When laying out regulations for the Fellowship offering, God instructs in Lev. 3:14-17

> *"14 From what he (the priest) offers he is to make this offering to the Lord by fire: all the fat that covers the inner parts or is connected to them, 15 both kidneys with the fat on them near the loins, and the covering of the liver, which he will remove with the kidneys. 16The priest shall burn them on the altar as food, an offering made by fire, a pleasing aroma. <u>All the fat is the Lord's</u>. 17This is a lasting ordinance for the generations to come, wherever you live. You must not eat any fat or blood."*

An appropriate passage of scripture to show the literal manifestation of this ordinance coming to life before us is found in 1 Samuel 2:12-16 where Hophni and Phinehas, sons of the priest, Eli, (specifically identified by name later in verse 34) set themselves up for a death sentence from God, partly because of their disobedience involving the Lord's ordinance regarding fat:

> [12]*"Eli's sons were wicked men; they had no regard for the Lord.* [13]*Now it was the practice of the priests with the people that whenever anyone offered a sacrifice and while the meat was being boiled, the servant of the priest would come with a three-pronged fork in his hand.* [14]*He would plunge it into the pan or kettle or caldron or pot, and the priest would take for himself whatever the fork brought up. This is how they treated all the Israelites who came to Shiloh.* [15]**But even before the fat was burned** *the servant of the priest would come and say to the man who was sacrificing, "Give the priest some meat to roast; he won't accept boiled meat from you but only raw."* [16] *If the man said to him, "Let the fat be burned up first, and then take whatever you want", the servant would then answer, "No hand it over now; if you don't I'll take it by force."* [17]*This sin of the young men was very great*

in the Lord's sight, for they were treating the
Lord's offering with contempt.

Remember that the fat of any meat is to be burned as a pleasing aroma to God and is not for our consumption. The scripture goes on to reveal that Eli, the priest, was warned about this grievous disregard and other sinful acts by his sons, but failed to deal with them firmly and effectively. Also remember that as priest, Eli would have been eating the very same fat-laden meat that his sons regularly brought to him. It should come as no surprise, then, that upon hearing the news about God making good on his promise to kill his two sons, Eli fell off his chair, broke his neck and died, too, because he was "an old man and *heavy*" (1 Samuel 4:18).

It should be very clear then, that when we prepare meat, it should be cooked long enough to render the fat out of it. The fat belongs to the Lord! If some lands on our plate anyway, we should trim it away and leave it!

When God finished His detailed regulations about clean and unclean food, He went on to do the same with what I believe is the foundation for sound practices still regarded today relative to infectious diseases and mildew (Lev. 13 and 14), sanitary practices surrounding bodily discharges (Lev. 15), sexual relations and various laws, which were more succinctly stated in what we now refer to as the Ten Commandments

(Lev. 19). In verse 37 of Leviticus 19, God made an encompassing statement:

> "Keep all my decrees and all my laws and follow them. I am the Lord."

He repeats this in chapter 20, verse 22-26.

> "Keep all my decrees and laws and follow them so that the land where I am bringing you to live may not vomit you out. You must not live according to the customs of the nations I am going to drive out before you. Because they did all these things, I abhorred them."

Abhor is a pretty strong word and emotion that the Lord expresses with regard to common practices that run counter to His decrees and laws! Through Moses, God then finished laying out the remainder of His decrees and laws, some of which was confirmed as being 'shadows and types' (in other words, regulations and decrees that God wanted to use to develop a code for holy living and establishing a framework for obedience, while giving us a 'shadow of life after the coming of the supreme sacrifice, Jesus Christ. It is important, then, to determine what of God's code for living was 'types and shadows' and, what was 'lasting ordinance' (surviving beyond the coming of Christ).

I think it is fairly well established (and there will be more on this later) that at least some of His commandments were not exclusive to Jews, nor limited to the Old Testament times. As pointed out here, specifically some of the dietary laws were identified as 'lasting ordinance'. To further support the relevance of God's laws for us (non-Jews), we should look to Isaiah 56:3:

> "Let no foreigner who has bound himself to the Lord say, "The Lord will surely exclude me from his people." And let no eunuch complain, I am only a dry tree."

In essence, **we who claim to be the Lord's people should not seek to exclude ourselves from His rules for holy living when we find them to be inconvenient.** To the contrary, knowing that they are for our own well-being, we should be quick and more than willing to embrace them. Even if it were true that these ordinances were only for the Jews, why would we not want them for ourselves, given the rewards God offers for obedience to them?

A little further in the book of Isaiah (chapter 65:2-5), we get a very graphic depiction of how God feels about pork consumption.

> "[2]All day long I have held out my hands to an obstinate people, who walk in ways not good, pursuing their own imaginations [3]a people who continually provoke me to my very face,. . . [4b] who eat the flesh of pigs,

and whose pots hold broth of unclean meat;
⁵who say, 'Keep away; don't come near me,
for I am too sacred for you!' Such people are
smoke in my nostrils, a fire that keeps burn-
ing all day."

(I don't think the Lord will be endorsing pork as the 'other white meat!!!) He goes on to say through Isaiah in verse 6, *"See, it stands written before me: I will not keep silent but will pay back in full; I will pay it back into their laps – both your sins and the sins of your fathers"*, says the Lord.

This word from Isaiah came literally hundreds of years after Moses and it is clear that God hadn't changed his mind about his laws. But, apparently his people had already done so, and yet again, strayed far from His ways.

In the last of his prophetic messages to us regarding the final judgment in chapter 66, verse 17, Isaiah proclaims,

"Those who consecrate and purify themselves
to go into the gardens, following the one in
the midst of those who eat the flesh of pigs
and rats and other abominable things – they
will meet their end together", *declares the*
Lord.

In John 15:1-17, Jesus himself (a Jew by the way) gives a brief discourse about the vine (native born

Jews) and the branches (Gentile Christians). In the middle of this passage in verse 10, Jesus states *"If you obey my commands, you will remain in my love, just as I have obeyed my Father's commands and remain in his love."* This concept of us as Gentiles being grafted in and treated as equals to native-born Israelites is presented yet again by Paul in Romans 11: 1-21. We should at the very least now be raising an eyebrow to accept as truth the continued relevance of God's word to professing Christians today.

I simply must particularly note verses 9 and 10 of the same 11th chapter of Romans, where Paul quotes David from Psalm 69:22-23 – *"May their table become a snare and a trap, a stumbling block and a retribution for them. May their eyes be darkened so they cannot see, and their backs be bent forever."*

I am certainly not trying to force the notion of that being pertinent to our questions about diet, but it clearly could fit to address those who are disobedient to God's laws with respect to His commands regarding clean and unclean food. In actuality, though it is preceded by David's pronouncement about his enemies, saying in verse 21 of Psalm 69, "They put gall in my food and gave me vinegar for my thirst." So, the two verses that follow really do literally make reference to food and what can happen if other than 'good' food is consumed (eyes darkened or blindness and bent backs or feebleness).

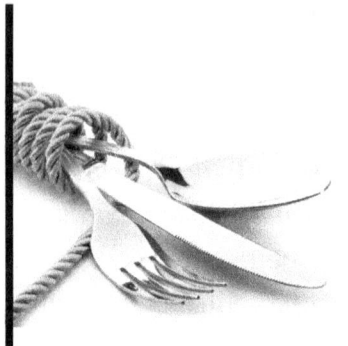

WHY SICKNESS AND DISEASE?

Why is there sickness and disease?
Why does God allow them?

Of course, there are many reasons for diseases and afflictions, ranging from sin and disobedience to less apparent ones passed off as mere chance or 'bad luck', fate and a host of other explanations, but what does God's word say? Proverbs 26:2 declares that *"an undeserved curse does not come to rest."* Notice the operative word, *undeserved*. Does this mean, then, that every person afflicted with illness deserves it? Absolutely not! To confirm this, we need to look no further than the account of God's faithful servant, Job. He, a righteous man, was allowed to be afflicted to the very point of death to test his faithfulness to God. All in the course of a day, all of his children were killed and all of his worldly possessions were destroyed. Immediately following, his physical body was afflicted with boils and sores so badly that he could only find temporary relief by scraping himself with a sharp stone. His three best friends (after sitting with him silently for several days of not knowing what to say or do) suggested that his calamity was so severe that he must have had un-confessed sin in his life and he needed to repent in order to break the curse. Even Job's wife concluded and pronounced to him that he should just curse God and die! In spite of all that, Job persisted (truthfully) that he had not sinned and he continued to trust God through the entire ordeal. He announced to those present that even if God chose to kill him, he would continue to serve Him. Because of his unwavering loyalty, God returned all that Job had lost and gave him many more years as a bonus.

Job's experience was not at all because of sin, but a lesson from God of how we all can be tested and the rewards for remaining faithful through adversity.

So then, it may be fair to say that, although there can be others, God allows sickness to come upon us for mainly one of two reasons – to test our faith, or as a consequence of disobedience – either direct or generational.

For the purposes of this writing, I will keep references relative to sickness related to the matter at hand, food choices.

The Lord tells us the consequences of disobedience in Leviticus 26:14-16:

> *"But if you will not listen to me and carry out all these commands, and if you reject my decrees and abhor my commands and so violate my covenant, then I will do this to you: I will bring upon you sudden terror, wasting diseases and fever that will destroy your sight and drain away your life."*

Though I am taking the liberty to speculate just a little here, I feel it is safe to do so. I believe that 'wasting disease' and the draining away of life are synonymous with what we now call cancer, a term that did not exist at the time. However, those are certainly characteristics of what cancer does to the body as it progresses through its various stages. Radical cells eat away at the body from the inside out. When all treatment efforts no longer work or have failed, the cancerous cells cause the person to lose weight and deteriorate to the point where organs fail one-by-one until their life is all gone. What a dreaded sentence! The Lord further warns in verse 21,

> *" If you remain hostile to me and refuse to listen to me, I will multiply your afflictions seven times over, as your sins deserve."*
> Continuing in verse 23, *"If, in spite of these things you do not accept my correction, but*

continue to be hostile toward me, I myself will be hostile toward you and will afflict you for your sins seven times over."

How often have we seen cancer patients who seem to have won the battle through chemotherapy and/or radiation, only to find that months, even years later, the cancer returns. In most of those cases, there is nothing that can be done short of divine intervention. I can only wonder if it is because they returned to the unhealthy habits that caused the cancer in the beginning. But God, in his sovereignty and supreme justice not only metes out punishment for disobedience, but also rewards our obedience. Earlier in the same 26th chapter of Leviticus, God promises,

"If you follow my decrees and are careful to obey my commands, I will ...."

God then goes on to list a plethora of wonderful blessings to be realized by those who are obedient to His laws and decrees, among them, prosperity and long life.

We should also look to Deuteronomy 5:33 –

"Walk in the way that the Lord your God has commanded you, so that you may live and prosper and prolong your days in the land that you will possess."

That latter part of the verse confirms that God wants us to be blessed while we're here on earth, not to just spend the entirety of our days here waiting for the glory of heaven. However, those blessings are <u>conditional,</u> based upon our obedience to all of his commands, which are explicitly and repeatedly given in the Old Testament. After restating His decrees, laws and regulations from Leviticus in the book of Deuteronomy, the Lord declared through Moses in Deuteronomy 26:16-19,

> *"16The Lord your God commands you this day to follow these decrees and laws; carefully observe them with all your heart and with all your soul. 17You have declared this day that the Lord is your God and that you will walk in all His ways, that you will keep His decrees, commands and laws, and that you will obey Him. 18And the Lord has declared this day that you are His people, his treasured possession as He promised, and that you are to keep all His commands. 19He has declared that He will set you in praise, fame and honor high above all the nations He has made and that you will be a people holy to the Lord your God, as He has promised."*

A fair question to pose for pondering here is, **At what point did God alter the terms of our covenant relationship with Him such that we are no longer**

expected to keep our part but can still expect that He will honor His part?

I firmly believe that if we are faithful to uphold our end of the covenant as best we can, God, in His grace and mercy can and will protect and heal us from attacks on our health that come from sources outside of our control. This is supported in God's promise to believers in Mark 16:18,

> "… when they drink deadly poison, it will not hurt them at all …"

Of course, it is to be assumed that this is referring to those times when we encounter harmful agents unknowingly, not brashly flaunting and exploiting God's protection because we are His special people. As stated earlier, I would also like to reiterate that believing means that we have not only accepted His Word as truth, but have also aligned our actions with the Word. Then, we can expect Him to fulfill His promise of protection.

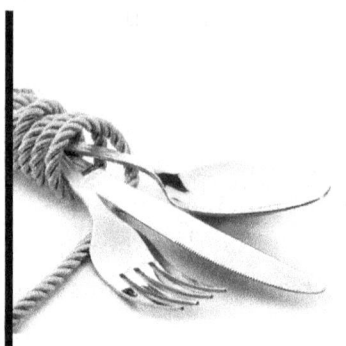

WHEN GOD DOESN'T HEAL

Why does God not cure people, even devout Christians, of cancer (and other terminal illnesses) when fervent prayers from strong, faith-filled believers are offered up on their behalf?

This is one of the most difficult questions to respond to, not because the answers are so elusive, but because nobody, including me, wants to be perceived as uncaring or insensitive when attempting to respond. Of course, a good and easy 'church' answer is "Well, God is sovereign and He can do whatever He wants. Sometimes it is just not His will to heal". Yes, God is sovereign and He can very well do whatever He chooses. But, let's focus for a moment on a more difficult, but valid response to offer, specifically relative to infirmities that are linked to wrong dietary choices. **"God has already given us His Word and instructions, as well as what to expect when we violate them. To heal ('so and so') in spite of their continued and willful disobedience of His commands and instructions would then be in violation of Himself and His word."** God cannot and will not do that – unless *"my people who are called by my name will humble themselves **and** pray **and** seek my face **and** turn from their wicked ways, **then** will I hear from heaven and will forgive their sins and will heal (their land). –* 2 Chronicles 7:14

I just learned recently of a fresh example of this awesome grace being extended to a local airline pilot. For the sake of anonymity, let's call him Mike. A few years ago, Mike was diagnosed with an aggressive form of cancer. The treatment and the devastating effects of the cancer itself rendered him disabled and unable to continue his duties as a pilot for a period of about two years. As so many have experienced before, doctors gave Mike the dreaded news that there was not much more they could do for him and he didn't have much longer to live. His major organs had begun to fail. Fortunately, Mike is a Christian and a fighter. During his time of debilitation, he studied the Bible intensely, using the Word to find and hold on to whatever measure of hope he could muster to cling to life. In so doing, he entered that proverbial 'room' mentioned in the earlier part of this book that most either never go into at all or they just peruse and keep going – that is the subject of God's dietary laws. As a result, Mike made immediate and major changes to how and what he ate. He prayed fervently and most importantly, he repented! Glory be to God!!! Mike has been healed and the cancer is gone! He is now teaching others in his Sunday school class the things he has learned and the power of God's word is touching their lives as well.

So, as you can see from 'Mike's' experience, through true repentance, there is the possibility of a pardon from a "Death Sentence for Dietary Disobedience". In His love, mercy and grace, God gives us a path back from our sin and disobedience. Yet, we often forget that *His love is unconditional, but His promises are not!* They require us to choose to do things differently. We cannot and should not expect God to contradict Himself and His Word, no matter how hard we pray, if we are not willing to meet all of His conditions. That is, if we knowingly or even out of ignorance will just return to the very same behaviors that got us in the shape we are in.

I am aware that there are countless testimonies of divine healing from cancer and many other diseases as a result of fervent prayer. In His sovereignty and omnipotence, God may certainly have done so for His glory and His purposes. After all, he even used a donkey to speak to Balaam (Numbers 22:28)! It wouldn't, then, be at all out of the question for Him to use a (albeit disobedient) human to glorify His name and accomplish a greater purpose. That having been said, that possibility does not in any way justify a total disregard for His laws on our part. Quite to the contrary, we should be committed, even overjoyed to willingly follow His leading. Out of His great love for us, those laws are only there for our good.

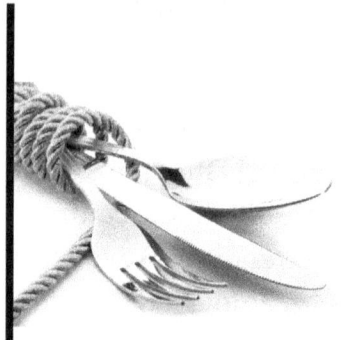

SIN OR JUST A MATTER OF CHOICE?

Is it a sin to eat so called "forbidden foods"?

This is unquestionably the most difficult of the questions posed that must be answered, not because the answer was particularly difficult to find, but because my honest response flies in the face of the widespread belief that the answer is, No.

Obviously, any who feel that what has been declared by God to be unclean is acceptable, would also feel that there is no sin in consuming the same. On far too many occasions, I have heard jokes (even from the pulpit) that doing so won't keep you out of heaven at all. If anything, it'll just get you there quicker! - makes for a good laugh, but if it really is sinful, it is certainly no laughing matter. Willful sin not only leads to death, but an eternal death! Scripture teaches us in Hebrews 10:26 that

> *"If we deliberately keep on sinning after we have received the knowledge of the truth, no sacrifice for sins is left,"*

So, you see, making the right call on this question is a matter of eternal life or death. Of course, the same applies to any area of our lives, not just what we choose to eat.

First, let's remember and consider that **the very first sin ever committed involved disobedience over what God had said was forbidden food.** In Genesis 2:17, God forbade Adam and Eve from eating from the Tree of Knowledge of Good and Evil.

Much like the animals He identified as unfit for human consumption, its being forbidden in no way determined it to be unpleasant to taste or in visual appeal (Genesis 2:9). We see this again in chapter 3, verse 6:

> ⁶ *When the woman saw that the fruit of the tree was good for food and pleasing to the eye, and also desirable for gaining wisdom, she took some and ate it. She also gave some to her husband, who was with her, and he ate it.*

That act of sin and disobedience introduced certain death to all of us, the only remedy being acceptance of the atoning blood of Christ.

Satan, appearing as a serpent, deceived Eve by twisting the facts and causing her to doubt God's words. Eve then proceeded to feed the forbidden fruit to Adam and he joined her in her sin. Had that fruit not been pleasing to the eye and to Eve's taste buds, Adam would not have likely been so tempted to partake.

Also, had God's warning of certain death been realized immediately, Adam (after watching Eve die and getting some answers from the Lord about why that happened) would probably have pleaded for a replacement companion and our fate might be very different today! However, just as it remains today, the consequence of eating forbidden food was not immediate. It may take years, even decades, for the cumulative effect of dietary disobedience to manifest as disease, infirmity or the like. In many cases, it may never become evident during the person's life here on earth. Herein lies the very reason I feel that **this area of spiritual discipline might be Satan's most effective stronghold on the people of God.** While we focus on the more obvious transgressions like sexual immorality, substance abuse, violence, theft, etc., **the enemy continues to pick us off one by one and in large numbers because we have rejected the truth of God's word on this subject.** In actuality, by being disobedient in the dietary laws, we unwittingly step outside of God's promised protection and play Russian Roulette with both our physical and spiritual lives nearly every time we sit down to a meal. We never know at what point we will get that dreaded news from the doctor about something that showed up in the blood or on the imaging exam.

OK, so perhaps you are the proverbial skeptic or an absolutist and you're saying "Alright, I get all that, but the Bible didn't really say that it was a sin – the word, sin, doesn't appear in this context".

You're right. It doesn't. However, it all comes together with unquestionable clarity when we read Romans 5:12, where Paul teaches, **"Sin entered the world through the one man (Adam) and death through sin . . . "**

So, you see, when God says, "do not" and we 'do', that is disobedience and disobedience is sin! It would be nice if that could be said in a more palatable way, but we are better served in the end to call it what it is and act accordingly.

As you have now read (hopefully) in such great detail God's commands and regulations regarding food and the fact that we *must choose* between the clean and the unclean, it should be crystal clear that your choices are not merely a matter of what you believe. Instead, they are a matter of sin or righteousness, life or death.

If, in spite of all that you have now read, you are still holding out and rationalizing to the effect of; "Well, after all, it's my body and I'm not hurting anyone else by what I choose to eat", think again! Assuming that you are a Christian, the following (1 Corinthians 6:19-20) applies to you:

> *¹⁹Do you not know that your body is a temple of the Holy Spirit, who is in you, whom you have received from God? You are not your own; ²⁰you were bought at a price. Therefore honor God with your body.*

Just a bit earlier in chapter 3, verse 17 the Word warns:

> *¹⁷If anyone destroys God's temple, God will destroy him; for God's temple is sacred, and you are that temple.*

I may be running the risk of overstating the obvious, but **when we accepted Christ, the Holy Spirit moved into our body and took up residence,** housed in a tabernacle (or temple) of flesh. **We then assumed an even greater responsibility to care for that temple.** We should make every effort to make sure that it is optimally fit to carry that same Holy Spirit and to maximize His ability to work in and through us. We are told in John 10:10 that Jesus desires that we have life (not 'stuff') and that more abundantly. That simply cannot most effectively be achieved if we are infirmed or impaired due to our own lack of discipline and poor choices.

At this point, I feel it is important to address an extremely important question that must be looming in the mind of many of you reading this material: "What about the countless Christians who have already passed on and they honestly did not know all of what was just read?" My response is multi-faceted. First, as a backdrop, it is important to be reminded of Hosea's prophetic statement (Hosea 4:6), "*my people are destroyed from lack of knowledge.*" Though this short passage of scripture has been used in myriads of contexts to support as many points, it is certainly fitting for this context. The information in this book is among much of scripture that countless saints who have passed on simply did not get or grasp. Right away, let's acknowledge that through the prophet, Hosea, God calls them **my** people, suggesting that He still regards those departed saints as his own. God makes allowances for ignorance, looking rather at the heart of the person and how they live based upon what they do know.

Here is where it gets a bit tricky. **To what extent does God's grace extend to those who conveniently avoid those biblical topics with which they are uncomfortable or do not agree?** How about those who only take in scripture when they attend church or listen to a sermon, never cracking their Bible (if they have one) to 'study to show themselves approved'? I will not pretend to possess the wisdom to conclusively answer those questions, but it certainly does seems a bit awry to expect to receive God's promises and benefits while being half-hearted in seeking Him, learning of His ways and applying them to our everyday lives. Nevertheless, I believe that there are those departed believers who earnestly lived according to the limited knowledge they had at the time, and the Lord will have mercy upon them and they will be enlightened to the truth as they enter into eternity with Him. On the other hand, I would not want to be among those who knew, but rejected that knowledge in favor of continuing in their own way rather than repenting and choosing to follow God's complete and perfect plan.

I desperately hope that I have presented the heart of God on this subject accurately and effectively enough to cause you to consider changes in your own dietary choices. I completely realize that this requires being quite different than most of the people around us, but we are supposed to come to know Jesus and to be a reflection of who He is. As such, we must also be obedient in every area of our lives. 1 John 2:3-4 puts it this way:

> *³We know that we have come to know him if we obey his commands. ⁴The man who says, "I know him," but does not do what he commands is a liar, and the truth is not in him.*

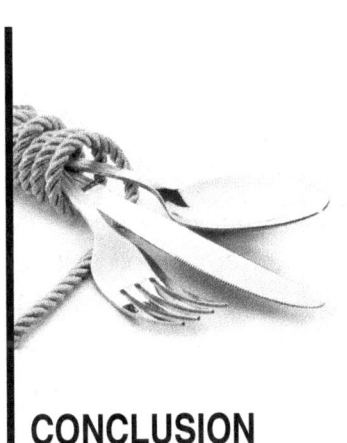

CONCLUSION

I am truly grateful for the time and effort you, the reader(s), have put forth to absorb this case for consideration of God's laws regarding our food choices. I repeat the acknowledgement that there are countless causes of illness and disease that are unrelated to willful violation of those laws. Some are environmental and some are caused by consumption of foods and beverages containing harmful agents that we are totally unaware of. However, as I said early on in this writing, I believe that our loving and merciful Father can and will protect and/or heal us from those things that are beyond our control when we are diligent and obedient in those areas that we know about and can control. In fact, I don't just believe it, I know it. To repeat 2 Chronicles 7:14,

> *"if my people, who are called by my name,*
> *will humble themselves and pray and seek my*

*face and turn from their wicked ways, **then**
will I hear from heaven and will forgive their
sin and will heal their land."*

Notice that this is a classic *'if/then'* conditional statement. Just like in mathematics, the end (*then*) result
will not come out right unless the *'if'* part is met **first.**
God stands ready to do just what He promises *if* you
will just do what He requires (first).

There is so much more that can be addressed in this
food choices arena, such as natural vs. artificial, sea
salt vs. table salt, natural sugar vs. refined sugar, etc.
There is also a vast amount of medical research and
scientific data available that establishes links between
common ailments and some of the very foods that God
labeled as unclean. However, for the sake of laying a
solid foundation, solely rooted in God's Word, they
are not included here. I am confident that the kingdom
of heaven and you will both be well served just by
implementing changes based on the material already
presented. And, as you are **turning** to God's dietary
plan and earnestly seeking to continue to grow in Him,
much of the additional information will be revealed to
you and confirmed valid by the Holy Spirit.

Yes, if you do decide that a change of dietary habits is in order for you, you will be required to give up
some of, perhaps, your favorite foods. I offer this as a
consolation: Remember that for every two *unclean* food

items you have to abandon, there are seven *clean* foods you can still enjoy!

In return for the time you have invested reading this, I pray that the Holy Spirit will reveal the truth to you. For any who are already experiencing the consequences of wrong choices made in ignorance, but are willing to repent and make better choices going forward, I pray with you and for you in the name of Jesus Christ, Yeshua, Messiah for God's grace and mercy and for a complete healing. I know that is possible, because He has done it many times before and He can do it for you! I thank Him for hearing and answering our prayer, bringing glory to His name!

May you be richly and abundantly blessed, both physically and spiritually. Amen.

In closing, I eagerly anticipate the return of testimonials of God's healing powers displayed as a result of changes made in the lives of those who read this book. This is not in any way because of any perceived prowess as a writer or special powers on my part, but a testament to my firm belief in God's faithfulness in honoring His Word.

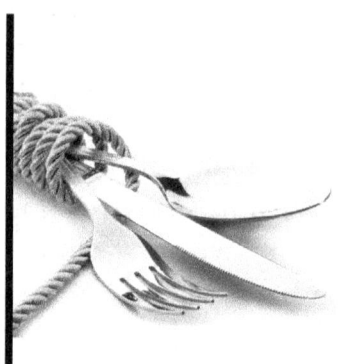

ABOUT THE AUTHOR

Don Harris is a student and highly regarded teacher of the Bible for more than twenty five years. He has been sought as a workshop speaker, clinician, public speaker and teacher. He is also a trained voice-over talent and welcomes new opportunities to utilize his gifts and talents to glorify God and enrich the lives of others. Don resides in the suburbs of Atlanta, GA and has been happily and faithfully married to Cynthia for 30 years.